First Aid

for

Caregivers

and

Babysitters

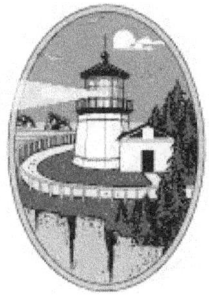

By

Charles Kennedy RN, LNHA

Contents

Contents

blank

Anaphylaxis:

A life-threatening allergic reaction (anaphylaxis) can cause shock, a sudden drop in blood pressure and trouble breathing. In people who have an allergy, anaphylaxis can occur minutes after exposure to a specific allergy-causing substance (allergen). In some cases, there may be a delayed reaction or anaphylaxis may occur without an apparent trigger.

If you're with someone having an allergic reaction with signs of anaphylaxis:

1. **Immediately call 911 or your local medical emergency number.**
2. Ask the person if he or she is carrying an epinephrine autoinjector to treat an allergic attack (for example, EpiPen, Twinject).
3. If the person says he or she needs to use an autoinjector, ask whether you should help inject the medication. This is usually done by pressing the autoinjector against the person's thigh.
4. Have the person lie still on his or her back.
5. Loosen tight clothing and cover the person with a blanket. Don't give the person anything to drink.
6. If there's vomiting or bleeding from the mouth, turn the person on his or her side to prevent choking.
7. If there are no signs of breathing, coughing or movement, begin CPR. Do uninterrupted chest presses of about two a second until paramedics arrive.
8. Get emergency treatment even if symptoms start to improve. After anaphylaxis, it's possible for symptoms to recur. Monitoring in a hospital setting for several hours is usually necessary.

If you're with someone having signs of anaphylaxis, don't wait to see whether symptoms get better. Seek emergency treatment right away. In severe cases, untreated anaphylaxis can lead to death within half an hour. An antihistamine pill, such as diphenhydramine (Benadryl, others), isn't sufficient to treat anaphylaxis. These medications can help relieve allergy symptoms, but work too slowly in a severe reaction to help.

Signs and symptoms of anaphylaxis include:

- Skin reactions including hives, itching, and flushed or pale skin

- Swelling of the face, eyes, lips or throat

- Constriction of the airways, leading to wheezing and trouble breathing

- A weak and rapid pulse

- Nausea, vomiting or diarrhea

- Dizziness, fainting or unconsciousness

Some common anaphylaxis triggers include:

- Medications (especially penicillin)

- Foods such as peanuts, tree nuts, fish and shellfish

- Insect stings from bees, yellow jackets, wasps, hornets and fire ants

If you've had any kind of severe allergic reaction in the past, ask your doctor if you should be prescribed an epinephrine autoinjector to carry with you.

Animal bites:

If an animal bites you or your family, follow these guidelines:

- **For minor wounds.** If the bite barely breaks the skin and there is no danger of rabies, treat it as a minor wound. Wash the wound thoroughly with soap and water. Apply an antibiotic cream to prevent infection and cover the bite with a clean bandage.

- **For deep wounds.** If the animal bite creates a deep puncture of the skin or the skin is badly torn and bleeding, apply pressure with a clean, dry cloth to stop the bleeding and see your doctor.

- **For infection.** If you notice signs of infection, such as swelling, redness, increased pain or oozing, see your doctor immediately.

- **For suspected rabies.** If you suspect the bite was caused by an animal that might carry rabies — including any wild or domestic animal of unknown immunization status — see your doctor immediately.

Doctors recommend getting a tetanus shot every 10 years. If your last one was more than five years ago and your wound is deep or dirty, your doctor may recommend a booster. You should have the booster as soon as possible after the injury.

Domestic pets cause most animal bites. Dogs are more likely to bite than cats are. Cat bites, however, are more likely to cause infection. Bites from nonimmunized domestic animals and wild animals carry the risk of rabies. Rabies is more common in raccoons, skunks, bats and foxes than in cats and dogs. Rabbits, squirrels and other rodents rarely carry rabies.

blank

10

Black eye:

The so-called black eye is caused by bleeding beneath the skin around the eye. Sometimes a black eye indicates a more extensive injury, even a skull fracture, particularly if the area around both eyes is bruised (raccoon eyes) or if there has been a head injury.

Although most black eye injuries aren't serious, sometimes there is an accompanying injury to the eyeball itself sufficient to cause bleeding inside the eye. Bleeding in the front part of the eye, called a hyphema, is serious and can reduce vision and damage the cornea — the clear, protective "window" at the front of the eye. In some cases, abnormally high pressure inside the eyeball (glaucoma) also can result. For this reason, it's advisable to have an eye specialist examine your eyeball if there has been enough of an injury to cause a black eye.

To take care of a black eye:

- Using gentle pressure, apply a cold pack or a cloth filled with ice to the area around the eye. Take care not to press on the eye itself. Apply cold as soon as possible after the injury to reduce swelling, and continue using ice or cold packs for 24 to 48 hours.

- Be sure there's no blood within the white and colored parts of the eye.

- Seek medical care immediately if you experience vision problems (double vision, blurring), severe pain, or bleeding in the eye or from the nose.

Blank

Bruise:

A bruise forms when a blow breaks blood vessels near your skin's surface, allowing a small amount of blood to leak into the tissues under your skin. The trapped blood appears as a black-and-blue mark.

If your skin isn't broken, you don't need a bandage, but you enhance bruise healing with these simple techniques:

- Elevate the injured area.

- Apply ice or a cold pack several times a day for a day or two after the injury.

- Rest the bruised area, if possible.

- Consider acetaminophen (Tylenol, others) for pain relief, or ibuprofen (Advil, Motrin, others) for pain relief and to reduce swelling.

See your doctor if:

- You have unusually large or painful bruises — particularly if your bruises seem to develop for no known reasons.

- You bruise easily and you're experiencing abnormal bleeding elsewhere, such as from your nose or gums, or you notice blood in your eyes, stool or urine.

- You have no history of bruising, but suddenly experience bruises.

These signs and symptoms may indicate a more serious problem, such as a blood-clotting problem or blood-related disease. Bruises accompanied by persistent pain or headache also may indicate a more serious underlying illness and require medical attention

Easy bruising: Common as you age

Find out what causes easy bruising as you age and when you should discuss your bruises with your doctor.

Yet another bruise. What caused that dark, unsightly mark on your leg? You don't recall bumping into anything. But lately you've been bruising much more often than you used to. Should you be concerned?

It's common to experience easy bruising with increasing age, and most bruises go away without treatment. Still, easy bruising can sometimes be a sign of a more serious problem.

Age-related causes of easy bruising in older adults

Most bruises form when small blood vessels (capillaries) near your skin's surface are broken by the impact of a blow or injury. When this happens, blood leaks out of the vessels and initially appears as a bright or dark red, purple or black mark. Eventually your body reabsorbs the blood, and the mark usually disappears.

Some people — especially women — are more prone to bruising than are others. As you get older, several factors may contribute to increased bruising, including:

- **Aging capillaries.** Over time, the tissues supporting these vessels weaken, and capillary walls become more fragile and prone to rupture.

- **Thinning skin.** With age, your skin becomes thinner and loses some of the protective fatty layer that helps cushion your blood vessels against injury. Excessive exposure to the sun accelerates the aging process in the skin.

Generally, the harder the blow, the larger the bruise. However, if you bruise easily, a minor bump — one you may not even notice — can result in substantial discoloration. Your arms and legs are typical locations for bruises.

Medications and supplements can cause easy bruising

Blood-thinning drugs such as aspirin and warfarin (Coumadin) or medications such as clopidogrel (Plavix) reduce your blood's ability to clot. Because of this, bleeding from capillary damage that would normally stop quickly may take longer to stop, allowing enough blood to leak out to cause a bruise.

Corticosteroids cause your skin to thin, making it easier to bruise. Don't stop taking your medications if you experience increased bruising. Talk to your doctor about your concerns and ask what you should do.

Certain dietary supplements such as fish oil and ginkgo also may increase your bruising risk, since these supplements have a blood-thinning effect. Make sure your doctor is aware of any supplements you're taking — especially if you're taking them while on a blood-thinning drug. Your doctor may recommend avoiding certain over-the-counter medications or supplements.

When bruises indicate more serious problems

Bruising may also indicate something more serious, such as a blood-clotting problem or a blood disease. See your doctor if:

- You have unusually large or painful bruises, particularly if your bruises seem to develop for no known reason

- You're bruising easily and you're experiencing abnormal bleeding elsewhere, such as from your nose, gums or intestinal tract

- You have no history of bruising but suddenly experience bruises, particularly if you recently started a new medication

These signs and symptoms can indicate that you have low levels — or abnormal function — of platelets, components of blood that help it clot after an injury. To diagnose the cause of your bruising, your doctor may check your blood platelet levels or do tests that measure the ability of your blood to coagulate.

Other serious causes of bruising include domestic violence or abuse. If a loved one has an unexplainable bruise, particularly in an unusual location such as around the eye or face, inquire about the possibility of abuse.

Avoiding bruises

Once a bruise has formed, not much can be done to treat it. Most eventually disappear as your body reabsorbs the blood.

If swelling is associated with the bruising, applying a cold compress for 20 minutes at a time and elevating the affected area may help. After the swelling has gone down, a warm compress may speed removal of the blood.

To prevent minor bruising, eliminate household clutter that could cause bumps or falls. Long-sleeved shirts and pants may provide an extra layer of protection for your skin. Avoid prolonged exposure to the sun to help you avoid its aging effects and the increased bruising risk that may result.

If the sight of your bruises bothers you, try covering them with makeup until they've healed.

Healing sequence and timeline

Bruises heal over approximately 72 hours to one week. Extensive bruising will take longer.

The stage of healing can be seen from the color change in the bruise:

Dark blue/purple (new) » blue » brown » green » yellow » healed

Burns:

To distinguish a minor burn from a serious burn, the first step is to determine the extent of damage to body tissues. The three burn classifications of **first-degree burn, second-degree burn and third-degree burn** will help you determine emergency care:

First-degree burn

The least serious burns are those in which only the outer layer of skin is burned, but not all the way through. The skin is usually red, with swelling, and pain sometimes is present. Treat a first-degree burn as a minor burn unless it involves substantial portions of the hands, feet, face, groin or buttocks, or a major joint, which requires emergency medical attention.

Second-degree burn

When the first layer of skin has been burned through and the second layer of skin (dermis) also is burned, the injury is called a second-degree burn. Blisters develop and the skin takes on an intensely reddened, splotchy appearance. Second-degree burns produce severe pain and swelling.

If the second-degree burn is no larger than 3 inches (7.6 centimeters) in diameter, treat it as a minor burn. If the burned area is larger or if the burn is on the hands, feet, face, groin or buttocks, or over a major joint, treat it as a major burn and get medical help immediately.

For minor burns, including first-degree burns and second-degree burns limited to an area no larger than 3 inches (7.6 centimeters) in diameter, take the following action:

- **Cool the burn.** Hold the burned area under cool (not cold) running water for 10 or 15 minutes or until the pain subsides. If this is impractical, immerse the burn in cool water or cool it with cold compresses. Cooling the burn reduces swelling by conducting heat away from the skin. Don't put ice on the burn.

- **Cover the burn with a sterile gauze bandage.** Don't use fluffy cotton, or other material that may get lint in the wound. Wrap the gauze loosely to avoid putting pressure on burned skin. Bandaging keeps air off the burn, reduces pain and protects blistered skin.

- **Take an over-the-counter pain reliever.** These include aspirin, ibuprofen (Advil, Motrin, others), naproxen (Aleve) or acetaminophen (Tylenol, others). Use caution when giving aspirin to children or teenagers. Though aspirin is approved for use in children older than age 2, children and teenagers recovering from chickenpox or flu-like symptoms should never take aspirin. Talk to your doctor if you have concerns.

Minor burns usually heal without further treatment. They may heal with pigment changes, meaning the healed area may be a different color from the surrounding skin. Watch for signs of infection, such as increased pain, redness, fever, swelling or oozing. If infection develops, seek medical help. Avoid re-injuring or tanning if the burns are less than a year old — doing so may cause more extensive pigmentation changes. Use sunscreen on the area for at least a year.

Caution

- **Don't use ice.** Putting ice directly on a burn can cause a burn victim's body to become too cold and cause further damage to the wound.

- **Don't apply butter or ointments to the burn.** This could cause infection.

- **Don't break blisters.** Broken blisters are more vulnerable to infection.

Third-degree burn
The most serious burns involve all layers of the skin and cause permanent tissue damage. Fat, muscle and even bone may be affected. Areas may be charred black or appear dry and white. Difficulty inhaling and exhaling, carbon monoxide poisoning, or other toxic effects may occur if smoke inhalation accompanies the burn.

For major burns, call 911 or emergency medical help. Until an emergency unit arrives, follow these steps:

1. **Don't remove burned clothing.** However, do make sure the victim is no longer in contact with smoldering materials or exposed to smoke or heat.

2. **Don't immerse large severe burns in cold water.** Doing so could cause a drop in body temperature (hypothermia) and deterioration of blood pressure and circulation (shock).

3. **Check for signs of circulation (breathing, coughing or movement).** If there is no breathing or other sign of circulation, begin CPR.

4. **Elevate the burned body part or parts.** Raise above heart level, when possible.

5. **Cover the area of the burn.** Use a cool, moist, sterile bandage; clean, moist cloth; or moist towels.

Get a tetanus shot. Burns are susceptible to tetanus. Doctors recommend you get a tetanus shot every 10 years. If your last shot was more than five years ago, your doctor may recommend a tetanus shot booster.

Chemical burns:

If a chemical burns the skin, follow these steps:

1. **Remove the cause of the burn** by first brushing any remaining dry chemical and then rinsing the chemical off the skin surface with cool, gently running water for 20 minutes or more.

2. **Remove clothing or jewelry** that has been contaminated by the chemical.

3. **Wrap the burned area loosely** with a dry, sterile dressing or a clean cloth.

4. **Rewash the burned area** for several more minutes if the person experiences increased burning after the initial washing.

5. **Take an over-the-counter pain reliever.** These include aspirin, ibuprofen (Advil, Motrin, others), naproxen (Aleve) or acetaminophen (Tylenol, others). Use caution when giving aspirin to children or teenagers. Though aspirin is approved for use in children older than age 2, children and teenagers recovering from chickenpox or flu-like symptoms should never take aspirin. Talk to your doctor if you have concerns.

Get a tetanus shot. All burns are susceptible to tetanus. Doctors recommend you get a tetanus shot every 10 years. If your last shot was more than five years ago, your doctor may recommend a tetanus shot booster.

Minor chemical burns usually heal without further treatment.

Seek emergency medical assistance if:

- The person shows signs of shock, such as fainting, pale complexion or breathing in a notably shallow manner

- The chemical burn penetrated through the first layer of skin, and the resulting second-degree burn covers an area more than 3 inches (7.6 centimeters) in diameter

- The chemical burn occurred on the eye, hands, feet, face, groin or buttocks, or over a major joint

- The person has pain that cannot be controlled with over-the-counter pain relievers

If you're unsure whether a substance is toxic,

call the poison control center at 800-222-1222.

If you seek emergency assistance, take the chemical container or a complete description of the substance with you for identification.

Chemical splash in the eye:

If a chemical splashes into your eye, take these steps immediately:
Flush your eye with water. Use clean, lukewarm tap water for at least 20 minutes, and use whichever of these approaches is quickest:

- Get into the shower and aim a gentle stream of lukewarm water on your forehead over your affected eye. Or direct the stream on the bridge of your nose if both eyes are affected. Hold your affected eye or eyes open.

- Put your head down and turn it to the side. Then hold your affected eye open under a gently running faucet.

- Young children may do best if they lie down in the bathtub or lean back over a sink while you pour a gentle stream of water on the forehead over the affected eye or on the bridge of the nose for both eyes.

Wash your hands with soap and water. Thoroughly rinse your hands to be sure no chemical or soap is left on them. Your first goal is to get the chemical off the surface of your eye, but then you must remove the chemical from your hands.

Remove contact lenses. If they don't come out during the flush, then take them out.

Caution:
- Don't rub the eye — this may cause further damage.

- Don't put anything except water or contact lens saline rinse in the eye, and don't use eyedrops unless emergency personnel tell you to do so.

Seek emergency medical assistance
After following the above steps, seek emergency care or, if necessary, call 911 or your local emergency number. Take the chemical container or the name of the chemical with you to the emergency department. If readily available, wear sunglasses because your eyes will be sensitive to light.

blank

Chest pain:

Causes of chest pain can vary from minor problems, such as indigestion or stress, to serious medical emergencies, such as a heart attack or pulmonary embolism. The specific cause of chest pain is often difficult to interpret.

Finding the cause of your chest pain can be challenging, especially if you've never had symptoms in the past. Even doctors may have a difficult time deciding if chest pain is a sign of a heart attack or something less serious, such as indigestion. If you have unexplained chest pain lasting more than a few minutes, you should seek emergency medical assistance rather than trying to diagnose the cause yourself.

As with other sudden, unexplained pains, chest pain may be a signal for you to get medical help. Use the following information to help you determine whether your chest pain is a medical emergency.

Heart attack

A heart attack occurs when an artery that supplies oxygen to your heart muscle becomes blocked. A heart attack may cause chest pain that lasts 15 minutes or longer. But a heart attack can also be silent and produce no signs or symptoms.

Many people who experience a heart attack have warning symptoms hours, days or weeks in advance. The earliest warning sign of an attack may be ongoing episodes of chest pain that start when you're physically active, but are relieved by rest.

Someone having a heart attack may experience any or all of the following:

- Uncomfortable pressure, fullness or squeezing pain in the center of the chest lasting more than a few minutes

- Pain spreading to the shoulders, neck or arms

- Lightheadedness, fainting, sweating, nausea or shortness of breath

If you or someone else may be having a heart attack:

- **Call 911 or emergency medical assistance.** Don't "tough out" the symptoms of a heart attack for more than five minutes. If you don't have access to emergency medical services, have someone, such as a neighbor or friend, drive you to the nearest hospital. Drive yourself only as a last resort, if there are absolutely no other options. Driving yourself puts you and others at risk if your condition suddenly worsens.

- **Chew a regular-strength aspirin.** Aspirin reduces blood clotting, which can help blood flow through a narrowed artery that's caused a heart attack. However, don't take aspirin if you are allergic to aspirin, have bleeding problems or take another blood-thinning medication, or if your doctor previously told you not to do so.

- **Take nitroglycerin, if prescribed.** If you think you're having a heart attack and your doctor has previously prescribed nitroglycerin for you, take it as directed. Don't take anyone else's nitroglycerin.

- **If the person is not breathing or does not have a pulse begin CPR**

Angina

Angina is a type of chest pain or discomfort caused by reduced blood flow to your heart muscle. Angina may be stable or unstable:

- Stable angina — persistent, recurring chest pain that usually occurs with exertion

- Unstable angina — sudden, new chest pain, or a change in the pattern of previously stable angina, that may signal an impending heart attack

Angina is relatively common, but can be hard to distinguish from other types of chest pain, such as the pain or discomfort of indigestion.

Angina signs and symptoms include:

- Chest pain or discomfort

- Pain in your arms, neck, jaw, shoulder or back accompanying chest pain

- Nausea

- Fatigue

- Shortness of breath

- Anxiety

- Sweating

- Dizziness

The severity, duration and type of angina can vary. If you have new or changing chest pain, these new or different symptoms may signal a more dangerous form of angina (unstable angina) or a heart attack. If your angina gets worse or changes, becoming unstable, seek medical attention immediately.

Pulmonary embolism

Pulmonary embolism occurs when a clot — usually from the veins of your leg or pelvis — lodges in an artery of your lung. The lung tissue served by the artery doesn't get enough blood flow, causing tissue death. This makes it more difficult for your lungs to provide oxygen to the rest of your body.

Signs and symptoms of pulmonary embolism include:

- Sudden, sharp chest pain that begins or worsens with a deep breath or a cough, often accompanied by shortness of breath

- Sudden, unexplained shortness of breath, even without pain

- Cough that may produce blood-streaked sputum

- Rapid heartbeat

- Fainting

- Anxiety

- Sweating

Pulmonary embolism can be life-threatening. As with a suspected heart attack, **call 911 or emergency medical assistance immediately.**

Aortic dissection

An aortic dissection is a serious condition in which a tear develops in the inner layer of the aorta, the large blood vessel branching off the heart. Blood surges through this tear into the middle layer of the aorta, causing the inner and middle layers to separate (dissect). If the blood-filled channel ruptures through the outside aortic wall, aortic dissection is usually fatal.

If you think aortic dissection is the cause of your chest pain, seek emergency medical assistance immediately.

Pneumonia with pleurisy

Frequent signs and symptoms of pneumonia are chest pain accompanied by chills, fever and a cough that may produce bloody or foul-smelling sputum. When pneumonia occurs with an inflammation of the membranes that surround the lung (pleura), you may have considerable chest discomfort when inhaling or coughing. This condition is called pleurisy.

One sign of pleurisy is that the pain is usually relieved temporarily by holding your breath or putting pressure on the painful area of your chest. This isn't true of a heart attack. If you've recently been diagnosed with pneumonia and then start having symptoms of pleurisy, contact your doctor or seek immediate medical attention to determine the cause of your chest pain. Pleurisy alone isn't a medical emergency, but you shouldn't try to make the diagnosis yourself.

Chest wall pain

One of the most common varieties of harmless chest pain is chest wall pain. One kind of chest wall pain is costochondritis. It causes pain and tenderness in and around the cartilage that connects your ribs to your breastbone (sternum).

In costochondritis, pressing on a few points along the edge of your sternum often results in considerable tenderness in those small areas. If the pressure of a finger causes similar chest pain, it's unlikely that a serious condition, such as a heart attack, is the cause of your chest pain.

Other causes of chest pain include:

- Strained chest muscles from overuse or excessive coughing

- Chest muscle bruising from minor injury

- Short-term, sudden anxiety with rapid breathing

- Peptic ulcer disease

- Pain from the digestive tract, such as esophageal reflux, peptic ulcer pain or gallbladder pain that may feel similar to heart attack symptoms

blank

Corneal abrasion (scratch):

The most common types of eye injury involve the cornea — the clear, protective "window" at the front of your eye. Contact with dust, dirt, sand, wood shavings, metal particles or even an edge of a piece of paper can scratch or cut the cornea. Usually the scratch is superficial, and this is called a corneal abrasion. Some corneal abrasions become infected and result in a corneal ulcer, which is a serious problem. Corneal abrasions caused by plant matter (such as a pine needle) can cause a delayed inflammation inside the eye (iritis).

Corneal abrasions can be painful. If your cornea is scratched, you might feel like you have sand in your eye. Tears, blurred vision, increased sensitivity or redness around the eye can suggest a corneal abrasion. You may get a headache.

In case of corneal abrasion, seek prompt medical attention. Other immediate steps you can take for a corneal abrasion are to:

- **Rinse your eye with clean water (use a saline solution, if available).** You can use an eyecup or small, clean drinking glass positioned with its rim resting on the bone at the base of your eye socket. If your work site has an eye-rinse station, use it. Rinsing the eye may wash out a foreign object.

- **Blink several times.** This movement may remove small particles of dust or sand.

- **Pull the upper eyelid over the lower eyelid.** The lashes of your lower eyelid can brush a foreign object from the undersurface of your upper eyelid.

Take caution to avoid certain actions that may aggravate the injury:

- **Don't try to remove an object** that's embedded in your eyeball. Also avoid trying to remove a large object that makes closing the eye difficult.

- **Don't rub your eye after an injury.** Touching or pressing on your eye can worsen a corneal abrasion.

- **Don't touch your eyeball** with cotton swabs, tweezers or other instruments. This can aggravate a corneal abrasion.

Dislocation:

A dislocation is an injury in which the ends of your bones are forced from their normal positions. The cause is usually trauma, such as a blow or fall, but dislocation can be caused by an underlying disease, such as rheumatoid arthritis.

Dislocations are common injuries in contact sports, such as football and hockey, and in sports that may involve falls, such as downhill skiing and volleyball. Dislocations may occur in major joints, such as your shoulder, hip, knee, elbow or ankle or in smaller joints, such as your finger, thumb or toe.

The injury will temporarily deform and immobilize your joint and may result in sudden and severe pain and swelling. A dislocation requires prompt medical attention to return your bones to their proper positions.

If you believe you have dislocated a joint:

1. **Don't delay medical care.** Get medical help immediately.
2. **Don't move the joint.** Until you receive help, splint the affected joint into its fixed position. Don't try to move a dislocated joint or force it back into place. This can damage the joint and its surrounding muscles, ligaments, nerves or blood vessels.
3. **Put ice on the injured joint.** This can help reduce swelling by controlling internal bleeding and the buildup of fluids in and around the injured joint.

blank

Electrical Injuries:

Electrical burns:

An electrical burn may appear minor or not show on the skin at all, but the damage can extend deep into the tissues beneath your skin. If a strong electrical current passes through your body, internal damage, such as a heart rhythm disturbance or cardiac arrest, can occur. Sometimes the jolt associated with the electrical burn can cause you to be thrown or to fall, resulting in fractures or other associated injuries.

Call 911 or your local emergency number for assistance if the person who has been burned is in pain, is confused, or is experiencing changes in his or her breathing, heartbeat or consciousness.

While helping someone with an electrical burn and waiting for medical help, follow these steps:

1. **Look first. Don't touch.** The person may still be in contact with the electrical source. Touching the person may pass the current through you.

2. **Turn off the source of electricity if possible.** If not, move the source away from both you and the injured person using a dry, nonconducting object made of cardboard, plastic or wood.

3. **Check for signs of circulation (breathing, coughing or movement).** If absent, begin cardiopulmonary resuscitation (CPR) immediately.

4. **Prevent shock.** Lay the person down with the head slightly lower than the trunk, if possible, and the legs elevated.

5. **Cover the affected areas.** If the person is breathing, cover any burned areas with a sterile gauze bandage, if available, or a clean cloth. Don't use a blanket or towel, because loose fibers can stick to the burns.

Electrical shock:

The danger from an electrical shock depends on the type of current, how high the voltage is, how the current traveled through the body, the person's overall health and how quickly the person is treated.

Call 911 or your local emergency number immediately if any of these signs or symptoms occur:

- Cardiac arrest

- Heart rhythm problems (arrhythmias)

- Respiratory failure

- Muscle pain and contractions

- Burns

- Seizures

- Numbness and tingling

- Unconsciousness

While waiting for medical help, follow these steps:

- **Look first. Don't touch.** The person may still be in contact with the electrical source. Touching the person may pass the current through you.

- **Turn off the source of electricity, if possible.** If not, move the source away from you and the person, using a nonconducting object made of cardboard, plastic or wood.

- **Check for signs of circulation (breathing, coughing or movement).** If absent, begin cardiopulmonary resuscitation (CPR) immediately.

- **Prevent shock.** Lay the person down and, if possible, position the head slightly lower than the trunk, with the legs elevated.

After coming into contact with electricity, the person should see a doctor to check for internal injuries, even if he or she has no obvious signs or symptoms.

Caution

- **Don't touch the person with your bare hands** if he or she is still in contact with the electrical current.

- **Don't get near high-voltage wires** until the power is turned off. Stay at least 20 feet away — farther if wires are jumping and sparking.

- **Don't move a person** with an electrical injury unless the person is in immediate danger.

blank

Fainting:

Fainting occurs when the blood supply to your brain is momentarily inadequate, causing you to lose consciousness. This loss of consciousness is usually brief.

Fainting can have no medical significance, or the cause can be a serious disorder. Therefore, treat loss of consciousness as a medical emergency until the signs and symptoms are relieved and the cause is known. Discuss recurrent fainting spells with your doctor.

If you feel faint:

- **Lie down or sit down.** To reduce the chance of fainting again, don't get up too quickly.

- **Place your head between your knees** if you sit down.

If someone else faints:

- **Position the person on his or her back.** If the person is breathing, restore blood flow to the brain by raising the person's legs above heart level — about 12 inches (30 centimeters) — if possible. Loosen belts, collars or other constrictive clothing. To reduce the chance of fainting again, don't get the person up too quickly. If the person doesn't regain consciousness within one minute, call 911 or your local emergency number.

- **Check the person's airway to be sure it's clear.** Watch for vomiting.

- **Check for signs of circulation (breathing, coughing or movement).** If absent, begin CPR. **Call 911** or your local emergency number. Continue CPR until help arrives or the person responds and begins to breathe.

If the person was injured in a fall associated with a faint, treat any bumps, bruises or cuts appropriately. Control bleeding with direct pressure.

Blank

Fever:

Fever is a sign of a variety of medical conditions, including infection. Your normal temperature may differ slightly from the average body temperature of 98.6 F (37 C).

For young children and infants, even slightly elevated temperatures may indicate a serious infection. In newborns, either a subnormal temperature or a fever may be a sign of serious illness. For adults, a fever usually isn't dangerous until it reaches 103 F (39.4 C) or higher.

Don't treat fevers below 102 F (38.9 C) with any medications unless your doctor tells you to. If you have a fever of 102 F (38.9 C) or higher, your doctor may suggest taking an over-the-counter medication, such as acetaminophen (Tylenol, others) or ibuprofen (Advil, Motrin, others).

Adults also may use aspirin, but don't give aspirin to children. It may trigger a rare, but potentially fatal, disorder known as Reye's syndrome. Also, don't give ibuprofen to infants younger than 6 months of age.

Fahrenheit-Celsius conversion table	
°F	°C
105	40.6
104	40.0
103	39.4
102	38.9
101	38.3
100	37.8
99	37.2
98	36.7
97	36.1
96	35.6

How to take a temperature

Today most thermometers have digital readouts. Some take the temperature quickly from the ear canal and can be especially useful for young children and older adults. Other thermometers can be used rectally, orally or under the arm.

If you use a digital thermometer, be sure to read the instructions so that you know what the beeps mean and when to read the thermometer. Under normal circumstances, temperatures tend to be highest around 4 p.m. and lowest around 4 a.m.

Because of the potential for mercury exposure or ingestion, glass mercury thermometers have been phased out and are no longer recommended.

Rectally (for infants)
To take your child's temperature rectally:

- Place a dab of petroleum jelly or other lubricant on the bulb.

- Lay your child on his or her stomach.

- Carefully insert the bulb one-half inch to one inch into the rectum.

- Hold the bulb and child still for three minutes. To avoid injury, don't let go of the thermometer while it's inside your child.

- Remove the thermometer and read the temperature as recommended by the manufacturer.

Taking a rectal temperature is also an option for older adults when taking an oral temperature is not possible.

A rectal temperature reading is generally 1 degree Fahrenheit (about 0.5 degree Celsius) higher than an oral reading.

Orally
To take your temperature orally:

- Place the bulb under your tongue

- Close your mouth for the recommended amount of time, usually three minutes

Under the arm (axillary)

Although it's not the most accurate way to take a temperature, you can also use an oral thermometer for an armpit reading:

- Place the thermometer under your arm with your arm down.

- Hold your arms across your chest.

- Wait five minutes or as recommended by your thermometer's manufacturer.

- Remove the thermometer and read the temperature.

To take your child's axillary temperature, have the child sit in your lap, facing to the side. Place the thermometer under your child's near arm, which should be against your chest.

An axillary reading is generally 1 degree Fahrenheit (about 0.5 degree Celsius) lower than an oral reading.

Get medical help for a fever if:

- A baby younger than 3 months has a rectal temperature of 100.4 F (38 C) or higher, even if your baby doesn't have other signs or symptoms

- A baby older than 3 months has a temperature of 102 F (38.9 C) or higher

- A newborn has a lower than normal temperature — less than 97 F (36.1 C) rectally

- A child younger than age 2 has a fever longer than one day, or a child age 2 or older has a fever longer than three days

- An adult has a temperature of more than 103 F (39.4 C) or has had a fever for more than three days

Call your doctor immediately if your child has a fever after being left in a hot car or if a child or adult has any of these signs or symptoms with a fever:

- A severe headache

- Severe swelling of the throat

- Unusual skin rash

- Unusual eye sensitivity to bright light

- A stiff neck and pain when the head is bent forward

- Mental confusion

- Persistent vomiting

- Difficulty breathing or chest pain

- Extreme listlessness or irritability

- Abdominal pain or pain when urinating

- Other unexplained symptoms

Food-borne illness:

All foods naturally contain small amounts of bacteria. But poor handling of food, improper cooking or inadequate storage can result in bacteria multiplying in large enough numbers to cause illness. Parasites, viruses, toxins and chemicals also can contaminate food and cause illness.

Signs and symptoms of food poisoning vary with the source of contamination, and whether you're dehydrated or have low blood pressure. Generally they include:

- Diarrhea

- Nausea

- Abdominal pain

- Vomiting (sometimes)

- Dehydration (sometimes)

With significant dehydration, you might feel:

- Lightheaded or faint, especially on standing

- Rapid heartbeat

Whether you become ill after eating contaminated food depends on the organism, the amount of exposure, your age and your health. High-risk groups include:

- **Older adults.** As you get older, your immune system may not respond as quickly and as effectively to infectious organisms as when you were younger.

- **Infants and young children.** Their immune systems haven't fully developed.

- **People with chronic diseases.** Having a chronic condition, such as diabetes or AIDS, or receiving chemotherapy or radiation therapy for cancer reduces your immune response.

If you develop food poisoning:

- Rest and drink plenty of liquids.

- Don't use anti-diarrheal medications because they may slow elimination of bacteria from your system.

Food-borne illness often improves on its own within 48 hours. Call your doctor if you feel ill for longer than two or three days or if blood appears in your stools.

Call 911 or call for emergency medical assistance if:

- You have severe symptoms, such as watery diarrhea that turns very bloody within 24 hours.

- You belong to a high-risk group.

- You suspect botulism poisoning. Botulism is a potentially fatal food poisoning that results from the ingestion of a toxin formed by certain spores in food. Botulism toxin is most often found in home-canned foods, especially green beans and tomatoes. Signs and symptoms of botulism usually begin 12 to 36 hours after eating the contaminated food and may include headache, blurred vision, muscle weakness and eventual paralysis. Some people also have nausea and vomiting, constipation, urinary retention, difficulty breathing, and dry mouth. These signs and symptoms require immediate medical attention.

Foreign objects :

Foreign object in the ear:

A foreign object in the ear can cause pain and hearing loss. Usually you know if an object is stuck in your ear, but small children may not be aware of it.

If an object becomes lodged in the ear, follow these steps:

- **Don't probe the ear with a tool.** Don't attempt to remove the foreign object by probing with a cotton swab, matchstick or any other tool. To do so is to risk pushing the object farther into the ear and damaging the fragile structures of the middle ear.

- **Remove the object if possible.** If the object is clearly visible, pliable and can be grasped easily with tweezers, gently remove it.

- **Try using gravity.** Tilt the head to the affected side to try to dislodge the object.

- **Try using oil for an insect.** If the foreign object is an insect, tilt the person's head so that the ear with the offending insect is upward. Try to float the insect out by pouring mineral oil, olive oil or baby oil into the ear. The oil should be warm but not hot. As you pour the oil, you can ease the entry of the oil by straightening the ear canal. Pull the earlobe gently backward and upward for an adult, backward and downward for a child. The insect should suffocate and may float out in the oil bath. Don't use oil to remove any object other than an insect. Do not use this method if there is any suspicion of a perforation in the eardrum — pain, bleeding or discharge from the ear.

If these methods fail or the person continues to experience pain in the ear, reduced hearing or a sensation of something lodged in the ear, seek medical assistance.

Foreign object in the eye:

If you get a foreign object in your eye:

- Wash your hands.

- Try to flush the object out of your eye with clean water or saline solution. Use an eyecup or a small, clean drinking glass positioned with its rim resting on the bone at the base of your eye socket.

To help someone else:

1. Wash your hands.
2. Seat the person in a well-lighted area.
3. Gently examine the eye to find the object. Pull the lower lid down and ask the person to look up. Then hold the upper lid while the person looks down.
4. If the object is floating in the tear film on the surface of the eye, try flushing it out with saline solution or clean, lukewarm water.

Caution

- Don't try to remove an object that's embedded in the eyeball.

- Don't rub the eye.

- Don't try to remove a large object that makes closing the eye difficult.

When to call for help
Call 911 or your local emergency number when:

- You can't remove the object.

- The object is embedded in the eyeball.

- The person with the object in the eye is experiencing abnormal vision.

- Pain, redness or the sensation of an object in the eye persists after the object is removed.

Foreign object in the nose:

If a foreign object becomes lodged in your nose:

- **Don't probe at the object** with a cotton swab or other tool.

- **Don't try to inhale the object** by forcefully breathing in. Instead, breathe through your mouth until the object is removed.

- **Blow out your nose gently** to try to free the object, but don't blow hard or repeatedly. If only one nostril is affected, close the opposite nostril by applying gentle pressure and then blow out gently through the affected nostril.

- **Gently remove the object** if it's visible and you can easily grasp it with tweezers. Don't try to remove an object that isn't visible or easily grasped.

- **Call for emergency medical assistance** or go to your local emergency room if these methods fail.

Foreign object in the skin:

If a foreign object is **projecting from** your skin:

- **Wash your hands and clean the area well** with soap and water.

- **Use tweezers** to remove splinters of wood or fiberglass, small pieces of glass or other foreign objects.

If the object is completely embedded in your skin:

Seek medical attention

Foreign object inhaled:

If you or your child inhales a foreign object, see your doctor. If the inhaled object causes choking, the American Red Cross recommends the **"five-and-five"** approach to delivering first aid:

- **First,** deliver five back blows between the victim's shoulder blades with the heel of your hand.

- **Next,** perform five abdominal thrusts (also known as the **Heimlich maneuver**).

- **Alternate** between five back blows and five abdominal thrusts until the blockage is dislodged.

If you're the only rescuer, perform back blows and abdominal thrusts before calling 911 or your local emergency number for help. If another person is available, have that person call for help while you perform first aid.

To perform the Heimlich maneuver on someone else:

- **Stand behind the person.** Wrap your arms around the waist. Tip the person forward slightly.

- **Make a fist with one hand.** Position it slightly above the person's navel.

- **Grasp the fist with the other hand.** Press hard into the abdomen with a quick, upward thrust — as if trying to lift the person up.

- **Perform a total of five abdominal thrusts**, if needed. If the blockage still isn't dislodged, repeat the five-and-five cycle.

To perform the Heimlich maneuver on yourself:

- **Place a fist** slightly above your navel.

- **Grasp your fist** with the other hand and bend over a hard surface — a countertop or chair will do.

- **Shove your fist** inward and upward.

Foreign object swallowed:

If you swallow a foreign object, it will usually pass through your digestive system uneventfully. But some objects can lodge in your esophagus, the tube that connects your throat and stomach. If an object is stuck in your esophagus, you may need to remove it, especially if it is:

- A pointed object, which should be removed as quickly as possible to avoid further injury to the esophageal lining

- A tiny watch- or calculator-type button battery, which can rapidly cause nearby tissue injury and should be removed from the esophagus without delay

If a swallowed object blocks the airway, the American Red Cross recommends the **"five-and-five"** approach to first aid:

- **First,** deliver five back blows between the victim's shoulder blades with the heel of your hand.

- **Next,** perform five abdominal thrusts (also known as the **Heimlich maneuver**).

- **Alternate** between five back blows and five abdominal thrusts until the blockage is dislodged.

Call 911 or your local emergency number for help.

Fractures (broken bones):

A fracture is a broken bone. It requires medical attention. If the broken bone is the result of major trauma or injury, **call 911 or your local emergency number. Also call for emergency help if:**

- The person is unresponsive, isn't breathing or isn't moving. Begin cardiopulmonary resuscitation (CPR) if there's no respiration or heartbeat.

- There is heavy bleeding.

- Even gentle pressure or movement causes pain.

- The limb or joint appears deformed.

- The bone has pierced the skin.

- The extremity of the injured arm or leg, such as a toe or finger, is numb or bluish at the tip.

- You suspect a bone is broken in the neck, head or back.

- You suspect a bone is broken in the hip, pelvis or upper leg (for example, the leg and foot turn outward abnormally).

Don't move the person except if necessary to avoid further injury. Take these actions immediately while waiting for medical help:

- **Stop any bleeding.** Apply pressure to the wound with a sterile bandage, a clean cloth or a clean piece of clothing.

- **Immobilize the injured area.** Don't try to realign the bone or push a bone that's sticking out back in. If you've been trained in how to splint and professional help isn't readily available, apply a splint to the area above and below the fracture sites. Padding the splints can help reduce discomfort.

- **Apply ice packs to limit swelling and help relieve pain until emergency personnel arrive.** Don't apply ice directly to the skin — wrap the ice in a towel, piece of cloth or some other material.

- **Treat for shock.** If the person feels faint or is breathing in short, rapid breaths, lay the person down with the head slightly lower than the trunk and, if possible, elevate the legs

Hip fracture

You can break your hip at any age, but the great majority of hip fractures occur in people older than 65. As you age, your bones slowly lose minerals and become less dense. Gradual loss of density weakens bones and makes them more susceptible to a hip fracture.

A hip fracture is a serious injury, particularly if you're older, and complications can be life-threatening. Fortunately, surgery to repair a hip fracture is usually very effective, although recovery often requires time and patience.

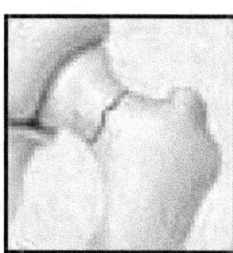

Signs and symptoms of a hip fracture include:

- Immobility immediately after a fall

- Severe pain in your hip or groin

- Inability to put weight on your leg on the side of your injured hip

- Stiffness, bruising and swelling in and around your hip area

- Shorter leg on the side of your injured hip

- Inward rotation of your leg on the side of your injured hip

Frostbite:

When exposed to very cold temperatures, skin and underlying tissues may freeze, resulting in frostbite. The areas most likely to be affected by frostbite are your hands, feet, nose and ears.

If your skin looks white or grayish-yellow, is very cold and has a hard or waxy feel, you may have frostbite. Your skin may also itch, burn or feel numb. Severe frostbite can cause blistering and hardening. As the area thaws, the flesh becomes red and painful.

Gradually warming the affected skin is key to treating frostbite. To do so:

- **Protect your skin from further exposure.** If you're outside, warm frostbitten hands by tucking them into your armpits. Protect your face, nose or ears by covering the area with dry, gloved hands. Don't rub the affected area and never rub snow on frostbitten skin.

- **Get out of the cold.** Once you're indoors, remove wet clothes.

- **Gradually warm frostbitten areas.** Put frostbitten hands or feet in warm water — 104 to 107.6 F (40 to 42 C). Wrap or cover other areas in a warm blanket. Don't use direct heat, such as a stove, heat lamp, fireplace or heating pad, because these can cause burns.

- **Don't walk on frostbitten feet or toes if possible.** This further damages the tissue.

- **If there's any chance the affected areas will freeze again, don't thaw them out.** If they're already thawed out, wrap them up so that they don't become frozen again.

- **Get emergency medical help.** If the skin turns red and there's a tingling and burning sensation as it warms, circulation is returning. But if numbness or sustained pain remains during warming or if blisters develop, seek medical attention.

blank

Head trauma:

Most head trauma involves injuries that are minor and don't require hospitalization. However, **call 911 or your local emergency number if any of the following signs or symptoms are apparent:**

- Severe head or facial bleeding

- Bleeding from the nose or ears

- Severe headache

- Change in level of consciousness for more than a few seconds

- Black-and-blue discoloration below the eyes or behind the ears

- Cessation of breathing

- Confusion

- Loss of balance

- Weakness or an inability to use an arm or leg

- Unequal pupil size

- Repeated vomiting

- Slurred speech

- Seizures

If severe head trauma occurs:

- **Keep the person still.** Until medical help arrives, keep the injured person lying down and quiet, with the head and shoulders slightly elevated. Don't move the person unless necessary, and avoid moving the person's neck.

- **Stop any bleeding.** Apply firm pressure to the wound with sterile gauze or a clean cloth. But don't apply direct pressure to the wound if you suspect a skull fracture.

- **Watch for changes in breathing and alertness.** If the person shows no signs of circulation (breathing, coughing or movement), begin CPR.

Heat Emergencies:

Heat cramps:

Heat cramps are painful, involuntary muscle spasms that usually occur during heavy exercise in hot environments. The spasms may be more intense and more prolonged than are typical nighttime leg cramps. Inadequate fluid intake often contributes to heat cramps.

Muscles most often affected include those of your calves, arms, abdominal wall and back, although heat cramps may involve any muscle group involved in exercise.

If you suspect heat cramps:

- Rest briefly and cool down

- Drink clear juice or an electrolyte-containing sports drink

- Practice gentle, range-of-motion stretching and gentle massage of the affected muscle group

- Don't resume strenuous activity for several hours or longer after heat cramps go away

- Call your doctor if your cramps don't go away within one hour or so

Heat exhaustion:

Heat exhaustion is one of the heat-related syndromes, which range in severity from mild heat cramps to heat exhaustion to potentially life-threatening heatstroke.

Signs and symptoms of heat exhaustion often begin suddenly, sometimes after excessive exercise, heavy perspiration, and inadequate fluid or salt intake. Signs and symptoms resemble those of shock and may include:

- Feeling faint or dizzy

- Nausea

- Heavy sweating

- Rapid, weak heartbeat

- Low blood pressure

- Cool, moist, pale skin

- Low-grade fever

- Heat cramps

- Headache

- Fatigue

- Dark-colored urine

If you suspect heat exhaustion:

- Get the person out of the sun and into a shady or air-conditioned location.

- Lay the person down and elevate the legs and feet slightly.

- Loosen or remove the person's clothing.

- Have the person drink cool water or other nonalcoholic beverage without caffeine.

- Cool the person by spraying or sponging him or her with cool water and fanning.

- Monitor the person carefully. Heat exhaustion can quickly become heatstroke.

If fever greater than 102 F (38.9 C), fainting, confusion or seizures occur, call 911 or emergency medical help.

Heatstroke:

Heatstroke is the most severe of the heat-related problems, seek medical attention immediately.

Often resulting from exercise or heavy work in hot environments combined with inadequate fluid intake.

Young children, older adults, people who are obese and people born with an impaired ability to sweat are at high risk of heatstroke. Other risk factors include dehydration, alcohol use, cardiovascular disease and certain medications.

What makes heatstroke severe and potentially life-threatening is that the body's normal mechanisms for dealing with heat stress, such as sweating and temperature control, are inadequate. The main sign of heatstroke is a markedly elevated body temperature — generally greater than 104 F (40 C) — with changes in mental status ranging from personality changes to confusion and coma. Skin may be hot and dry — although if heatstroke is caused by exertion, the skin may be moist.

Other signs and symptoms may include:
- Rapid heartbeat

- Rapid and shallow breathing

- Elevated or lowered blood pressure

- Cessation of sweating

- Irritability, confusion or unconsciousness

- Feeling dizzy or lightheaded

- Headache

- Nausea

- Fainting, which may be the first sign in older adults

If you suspect heatstroke:

- Move the person out of the sun and into a shady or air-conditioned space.

- **Call 911 or emergency medical help.**

- Cool the person by covering him or her with damp sheets or by spraying with cool water. Direct air onto the person with a fan or newspaper.

- Have the person drink cool water or other nonalcoholic beverage without caffeine, if he or she is able.

Hypothermia:

Under most conditions your body maintains a healthy temperature. However, when exposed to cold temperatures, especially with a high wind chill factor and high humidity, or to a cool, damp environment for prolonged periods, your body's control mechanisms may fail to keep your body temperature normal. When more heat is lost than your body can generate, hypothermia, defined as an internal body temperature less than 95 F (35 C), can result.

Wet or inadequate clothing, falling into cold water and even not covering your head during cold weather can increase your chances of hypothermia.

Signs and symptoms include:

- Shivering

- Slurred speech

- Abnormally slow breathing

- Cold, pale skin

- Loss of coordination

- Fatigue, lethargy or apathy

- Confusion or memory loss

- Bright red, cold skin (infants)

Signs and symptoms usually develop slowly. People with hypothermia typically experience gradual loss of mental acuity and physical ability, so they may be unaware that they need emergency medical treatment.

Older adults, infants, young children and people who are very lean are at particular risk. Other people at higher risk of hypothermia include those whose judgment may be impaired by mental illness or Alzheimer's disease and people who are intoxicated, homeless or caught in cold weather because their vehicles have broken down. Other conditions that may predispose people to hypothermia are malnutrition, cardiovascular disease and an underactive thyroid (hypothyroidism).

To care for someone with hypothermia:

- **Call 911 or emergency medical assistance.** While waiting for help to arrive, monitor the person's breathing. If breathing stops or seems dangerously slow or shallow, begin cardiopulmonary resuscitation (CPR) immediately.

- **Move the person out of the cold.** If going indoors isn't possible, protect the person from the wind, cover his or her head, and insulate his or her body from the cold ground.

- **Remove wet clothing.** Replace wet things with a warm, dry covering.

- **Don't apply direct heat.** Don't use hot water, a heating pad or a heating lamp to warm the victim. Instead, apply warm compresses to the center of the body — head, neck, chest wall and groin. Don't attempt to warm the arms and legs. Heat applied to the arms and legs forces cold blood back toward the heart, lungs and brain, causing the core body temperature to drop. This can be fatal.

- **Don't give the person alcohol.** Offer warm nonalcoholic drinks, unless the person is vomiting.

- **Don't massage or rub the person.** Handle people with hypothermia gently; their skin may be frostbitten, and rubbing frostbitten tissue can cause severe damage

Insect bites and stings:

Signs and symptoms of an insect bite result from the injection of venom or other substances into your skin. The venom sometimes triggers an allergic reaction. The severity of your reaction depends on your sensitivity to the insect venom or substance and whether you've been stung or bitten more than once.

Most reactions to insect bites are mild, causing little more than an annoying itching or stinging sensation and mild swelling that disappear within a day or so. A delayed reaction may cause fever, hives, painful joints and swollen glands. You might experience both the immediate and the delayed reactions from the same insect bite or sting. Only a small percentage of people develop severe reactions (anaphylaxis) to insect venom. Signs and symptoms of a severe reaction include:

- Nausea

- Facial swelling

- Difficulty breathing

- Abdominal pain

- Deterioration of blood pressure and circulation (shock)

Bites from bees, wasps, hornets, yellow jackets and fire ants are typically the most troublesome. Bites from mosquitoes, ticks, biting flies and some spiders also can cause reactions, but these are generally milder. Although rare, some insects also carry disease such as West Nile virus or Lyme disease.

For mild reactions

- **Move to a safe area** to avoid more stings.

- **Remove the stinger,** especially if it's stuck in your skin. This will prevent the release of more venom. Wash area with soap and water.

- **Apply a cold pack** or cloth filled with ice to reduce pain and swelling.

- **Apply hydrocortisone cream** (0.5 percent or 1 percent), calamine lotion or a baking soda paste — with a ratio of 3 teaspoons (15 milliliters) baking soda to 1 teaspoon (5 milliliters) water — to the bite or sting several times a day until symptoms subside.

- **Take an antihistamine** containing diphenhydramine (Benadryl, Tylenol Severe Allergy) or chlorpheniramine maleate (Chlor-Trimeton, Actifed).

Allergic reactions may include mild nausea and intestinal cramps, diarrhea, or swelling larger than 2 inches (5 centimeters) in diameter at the site. See your doctor promptly if you experience any of these signs and symptoms.

For severe reactions (anaphylaxis)

Severe reactions may progress rapidly. **Call 911 or emergency medical assistance if the following signs or symptoms occur:**

- Difficulty breathing

- Swelling of the lips or throat

- Faintness

- Dizziness

- Confusion

- Rapid heartbeat

- Hives

- Nausea, cramps and vomiting

Take these actions immediately while waiting with an affected person for medical help:

1. **Check for medications** that the person might be carrying to treat an allergic attack, such as an auto-injector of epinephrine (for example, EpiPen). Administer the drug as directed — usually by pressing the auto-injector against the person's thigh and holding it in place for several seconds. Massage the injection site for 10 seconds to enhance absorption.

2. **Have the person take an antihistamine pill** if he or she is able to do so without choking. Do this after administering epinephrine.

3. **Have the person lie still** on his or her back with feet higher than the head.

4. **Loosen tight clothing** and cover the person with a blanket. Don't give anything to drink.

5. **Turn the person on his or her side** to prevent choking if there's vomiting or bleeding from the mouth.

6. **Begin CPR** if there are no signs of circulation, such as breathing, coughing or movement.

If your doctor has prescribed an auto-injector of epinephrine, read the instructions before a problem develops and also have your household members read them.

blank

Nosebleeds:

Nosebleeds are common. Most often they are a nuisance and not a true medical problem. But they can be both.

Among children and young adults, nosebleeds usually originate from the septum, just inside the nose. The septum separates your nasal chambers.

In middle-aged and older adults, nosebleeds can begin from the septum, but they may also begin deeper in the nose's interior. This latter origin of nosebleed is much less common. It may be caused by hardened arteries or high blood pressure. These nosebleeds begin spontaneously and are often difficult to stop. They require a specialist's help.

To take care of a nosebleed:

- **Sit upright and lean forward.** By remaining upright, you reduce blood pressure in the veins of your nose. This discourages further bleeding. Sitting forward will help you avoid swallowing blood, which can irritate your stomach.

- **Pinch your nose.** Use your thumb and index finger to pinch your nostrils shut. Breathe through your mouth. Continue to pinch for five to 10 minutes. This maneuver sends pressure to the bleeding point on the nasal septum and often stops the flow of blood.

- **To prevent re-bleeding after bleeding has stopped,** don't pick or blow your nose and don't bend down until several hours after the bleeding episode. Keep your head higher than the level of your heart.

- **If re-bleeding occurs,** blow out forcefully to clear your nose of blood clots and spray both sides of your nose with a decongestant nasal spray containing oxymetazoline (Afrin, others). Pinch your nose in the technique described above and call your doctor.

Seek medical care immediately if:

- The bleeding lasts for more than 20 minutes

- The nosebleed follows an accident, a fall or an injury to your head, including a punch in the face that may have broken your nose

For frequent nosebleeds

If you experience frequent nosebleeds, make an appointment with your doctor. You may need a blood vessel cauterized. Cautery is a technique in which the blood vessel is burned with electric current, silver nitrate or a laser. Sometimes your doctor may pack your nose with special gauze or an inflatable latex balloon to put pressure on the blood vessel and stop the bleeding.

Also call your doctor if you are experiencing nasal bleeding and are taking blood thinners, such as aspirin or warfarin (Coumadin). Your doctor may advise adjusting your medication intake.

Using supplemental oxygen administered with a nasal tube (cannula) may increase your risk of nosebleeds. Apply a water-based lubricant to your nostrils and increase the humidity in your home to help relieve nasal bleeding.

Pink eye (conjunctivitis)

Pink eye (conjunctivitis) is an inflammation or infection of the transparent membrane (conjunctiva) that lines your eyelid and part of your eyeball. Inflammation causes small blood vessels in the conjunctiva to become more prominent, which is what causes the pink or red cast to the whites of your eyes.

The cause of pink eye is commonly a bacterial or viral infection, an allergic reaction or — in babies — an incompletely opened tear duct.

Though the inflammation of pink eye can be irritating, it rarely affects your vision. If you suspect pink eye, you can take steps to ease your discomfort. But because pink eye can be contagious, early diagnosis and treatment is best to help limit its spread.

Symptoms
The most common pink eye symptoms include:

- Redness in one or both eyes

- Itchiness in one or both eyes

- A gritty feeling in one or both eyes

- A discharge in one or both eyes that forms a crust during the night

- Tearing

When to see a doctor
Make an appointment with your doctor if you notice any signs or symptoms you think might be pink eye. Pink eye can be highly contagious for as long as two weeks after signs and symptoms begin. With an early diagnosis you can protect people around you from contracting pink eye, get treatment to help you cope with your symptoms and reduce your risk of complications.

Causes of pink eye include:

- Viruses

- Bacteria

- Allergies

- A chemical splash in the eye

- A foreign object in the eye

- In newborns, a blocked tear duct

Viral and bacterial conjunctivitis

Viral conjunctivitis and bacterial conjunctivitis may affect one or both eyes. Viral conjunctivitis usually produces a watery discharge. Bacterial conjunctivitis often produces a thicker, yellow-green discharge. Both viral and bacterial conjunctivitis can be associated with colds or with symptoms of a respiratory infection, such as a sore throat.

Both viral and bacterial types are very contagious. Adults and children alike can develop both of these types of pink eye. However, bacterial conjunctivitis is more common in children than it is in adults.

Allergic conjunctivitis

Allergic conjunctivitis affects both eyes and is a response to an allergy-causing substance such as pollen. In response to allergens, your body produces an antibody called immunoglobulin E (IgE). This antibody triggers special cells called mast cells in the mucous lining of your eyes and airways to release inflammatory substances, including histamines. Your body's release of histamine can produce a number of allergy signs and symptoms, including red or pink eyes.

If you have allergic conjunctivitis, you may experience intense itching, tearing and inflammation of the eyes — as well as sneezing and watery nasal discharge. Most allergic conjunctivitis can be controlled with allergy eyedrops.

Conjunctivitis resulting from irritation

Irritation from a chemical splash or foreign object in your eye is also associated with conjunctivitis. Sometimes, flushing and cleaning the eye to rid it of the chemical or object causes redness and irritation. Signs and symptoms, which may include watery eyes and a mucous discharge, usually clear up on their own within about a day.

Risk factors for pink eye include:

- Exposure to an allergen for allergic conjunctivitis

- Exposure to someone infected with the viral or bacterial form of conjunctivitis

- Using contact lenses, especially extended-wear lenses

Complications

In both children and adults, pink eye can cause inflammation in the cornea that can affect vision. Prompt evaluation and treatment by your doctor can reduce the risk of complications.

Preparing for your appointment

Start by seeing your family doctor or a general practitioner if you have any eye-related signs or symptoms that worry you. If your signs and symptoms persist or get worse, despite treatment, your doctor may refer you to an eye specialist (ophthalmologist).

Because appointments can be brief, and because there's often a lot of ground to cover, it's a good idea to be well prepared for your appointment. Here's some information to help you get ready for your appointment, and what to expect from your doctor.

What you can do

- **Be aware of any pre-appointment restrictions.** At the time you make the appointment, be sure to ask if there's anything you need to do in advance, such as stop wearing contact lenses or refrain from using eyedrops.

- **Write down any symptoms you're experiencing,** including any that may seem unrelated to the reason for which you scheduled the appointment.

- **Make a list of all medications,** as well as any vitamins or supplements, that you're taking.

- **Write down questions to ask** your doctor.

Your time with your doctor is limited, so preparing a list of questions can help you make the most of your time together. List your questions from most important to least important in case time runs out. For pink eye, some basic questions to ask your doctor include:

- What is likely causing my symptoms or condition?

- What are other possible causes for my symptoms or condition?

- What kinds of tests do I need?

- What is the best course of action?

- What are the alternatives to the primary approach that you're suggesting?

- I have these other health conditions. How can I best manage them together?

- Are there any restrictions that I need to follow?

- Should I see a specialist? What will that cost, and will my insurance cover it?

- Is there a generic alternative to the medicine you're prescribing me?

- Are there any brochures or other printed material that I can take with me? What Web sites do you recommend?

- What will determine whether I should plan for a follow-up visit?

What to expect from your doctor

Your doctor is likely to ask you a number of questions. Being ready to answer them may allow time later to cover points you want to address. Your doctor may ask:

- When did you begin experiencing symptoms?

- Have your symptoms been continuous or occasional?

- How severe are your symptoms?

- What, if anything, seems to improve your symptoms?

- What, if anything, appears to worsen your symptoms?

- Do your symptoms affect one eye or both eyes?

- Do you use contact lenses?

- How do you clean your contact lenses?

- How often do you replace your contact lens storage case?

- Have you had close contact with anyone who has pink eye or cold or flu symptoms?

Tests and diagnosis

To determine whether you have pink eye, your doctor may examine your eyes. Your doctor may also take a sample of eye secretions from your conjunctiva for laboratory analysis to determine which form of infection you have and how best to treat it.

Treatment for bacterial conjunctivitis

If your infection is bacterial, your doctor may prescribe antibiotic eyedrops as pink eye treatment, and the infection should go away within several days. Antibiotic eye ointment, in place of eye drops, is sometimes prescribed for treating bacterial pink eye in children. An ointment is often easier to administer to an infant or young child than are eyedrops, though the ointment may blur vision for up to 20 minutes after application. With either form of medication, expect signs and symptoms to subside within a few days. Follow your doctor's instructions and use the antibiotics until your prescription runs out, to prevent recurrence of the infection.

Treatment for viral conjunctivitis

There is no treatment for most cases of viral conjunctivitis. Instead, the virus needs time to run its course — up to two or three weeks. Viral conjunctivitis often begins in one eye and then infects the other eye within a few days. Your signs and symptoms should gradually clear on their own.

Antiviral medications may be an option if your doctor determines that your viral conjunctivitis is caused by the herpes simplex virus.

Treatment for allergic conjunctivitis

If the irritation is allergic conjunctivitis, your doctor may prescribe one of many different types of eye drops for people with allergies. These may include antihistamines, decongestants, mast cell stabilizers, steroids and anti-inflammatory drops. You may also reduce the severity of your of allergic conjunctivitis symptoms by avoiding whatever causes your allergies, when possible.

Poisoning:

Many conditions mimic the signs and symptoms of poisoning, including seizures, alcohol intoxication, stroke and insulin reaction. So look for the signs and symptoms listed below and if you suspect poisoning, call your regional poison control center or, in the United States, the **National Poison Control Center at 800-222-1222** before giving anything to the affected person.

Signs and symptoms of poisoning:

- Burns or redness around the mouth and lips, from drinking certain poisons

- Breath that smells like chemicals, such as gasoline or paint thinner

- Burns, stains and odors on the person, on his or her clothing, or on the furniture, floor, rugs or other objects in the surrounding area

- Empty medication bottles or scattered pills

- Vomiting, difficulty breathing, sleepiness, confusion or other unexpected signs

When to call for help:

Call 911 or your local emergency number immediately if the person is:
- Drowsy or unconscious

- Having difficulty breathing or has stopped breathing

- Uncontrollably restless or agitated

- Having seizures

If the person seems stable and has no symptoms, but you suspect poisoning, call your regional poison control center or, the **National Poison Control Center at 800-222-1222**.

Provide information about the person's symptoms, the person's age and weight, and any information you have about the poison, such as amount and how long since the person was exposed to it. It helps to have the pill bottle or poison container on hand when you call.

What to do while waiting for help:

- If the person has been exposed to poisonous fumes, such as carbon monoxide, get him or her into fresh air immediately.

- If the person swallowed the poison, remove anything remaining in the mouth.

- If the suspected poison is a household cleaner or other chemical, read the label and follow instructions for accidental poisoning. If the product is toxic, the label will likely advise you to call the poison control center at 800-222-1222. Also call this 800 number if you can't identify the poison, if it's medication or if there are no instructions.

- Follow treatment directions that are given by the poison control center.

- If the poison spilled on the person's clothing, skin or eyes, remove the clothing. Flush the skin or eyes with cool or lukewarm water, such as by using a shower for 20 minutes or until help arrives.

- Make sure the person is breathing. If not, start rescue breathing and CPR.

- Take the poison container (or any pill bottles) with you to the hospital.

What NOT to do

Don't give ipecac syrup or do anything to induce vomiting. The American Academy of Pediatrics advises discarding ipecac in the home, saying there's no good evidence of effectiveness and that it can do more harm than good.

Severe bleeding:

If possible, before you try to stop severe bleeding, wash your hands to avoid infection and put on synthetic gloves. Don't reposition displaced organs. If the wound is abdominal and organs have been displaced, don't try to push them back into place — cover the wound with a dressing.

For other cases of severe bleeding, follow these steps:

1. **Have the injured person lie down and cover the person to prevent loss of body heat.** If possible, position the person's head slightly lower than the trunk or elevate the legs. This position reduces the risk of fainting by increasing blood flow to the brain. If possible, elevate the site of bleeding.

2. **While wearing gloves, remove any obvious dirt or debris from the wound.** Don't remove any large or more deeply embedded objects. Don't probe the wound or attempt to clean it at this point. Your principal concern is to stop the bleeding.

3. **Apply pressure directly on the wound until the bleeding stops.** Use a sterile bandage or clean cloth and hold continuous pressure for at least 20 minutes without looking to see if the bleeding has stopped. Maintain pressure by binding the wound tightly with a bandage (or a piece of clean cloth) and adhesive tape. Use your hands if nothing else is available. If possible, wear rubber or latex gloves or use a clean plastic bag for protection.

4. **Don't remove the gauze or bandage.** If the bleeding continues and seeps through the gauze or other material you are holding on the wound, don't remove it. Instead, add more absorbent material on top of it.

5. **Squeeze a main artery if necessary.** If the bleeding doesn't stop with direct pressure, apply pressure to the artery delivering blood to the area of the wound. Pressure points of the arm are on the inside of the arm just above the elbow and just below the armpit. Pressure points of the leg are just behind the knee and in the groin. Squeeze the main artery in these areas against the bone. Keep your fingers flat. With your other hand, continue to exert pressure on the wound itself.

6. **Immobilize the injured body part once the bleeding has stopped.** Leave the bandages in place and get the injured person to the emergency room as soon as possible.

If you suspect internal bleeding, call **911 or your local emergency number**. Signs of internal bleeding may include:

- Bleeding from body cavities, such as the ears, nose, rectum or vagina

- Vomiting or coughing up blood

- Bruising on neck, chest, abdomen or side (between ribs and hip)

- Wounds that have penetrated the skull, chest or abdomen

- Abdominal tenderness, possibly accompanied by rigidity or spasm of abdominal muscles

- Fractures

- Shock, indicated by weakness, anxiety, thirst or skin that's cool to the touch

Shock:

Shock may result from trauma, heatstroke, blood loss, an allergic reaction, severe infection, poisoning, severe burns or other causes. When a person is in shock, his or her organs aren't getting enough blood or oxygen, which if untreated, can lead to permanent organ damage or death.

Various signs and symptoms appear in a person experiencing shock:

- **The skin is cool and clammy.** It may appear pale or gray.

- **The pulse is weak and rapid.** Breathing may be slow and shallow, or hyperventilation (rapid or deep breathing) may occur. Blood pressure is below normal.

- **The person may be nauseated.** He or she may vomit.

- **The eyes lack luster and may seem to stare.** Sometimes the pupils are dilated.

- **The person may be conscious or unconscious.** If conscious, the person may feel faint or be very weak or confused. Shock sometimes causes a person to become overly excited and anxious.

If you suspect shock, even if the person seems normal after an injury:

- **Call 911 or your local emergency number.**

- **Have the person lie down** on his or her back with feet about a foot higher than the head. If raising the legs will cause pain or further injury, keep him or her flat. Keep the person still.

- **Check for signs of circulation** (breathing, coughing or movement). If absent, begin CPR.

- **Keep the person warm and comfortable.** Loosen belt and tight clothing and cover the person with a blanket. Even if the person complains of thirst, give nothing by mouth.

- **Turn the person on his or her side** to prevent choking if the person vomits or bleeds from the mouth.

- **Seek treatment for injuries,** such as bleeding or broken bones.

Standard position for giving care for shock: feet up, injury elevated. Warning: Do not elevate the injury if you think a bone may be broken. Do not elevate *any* unsplinted fracture.

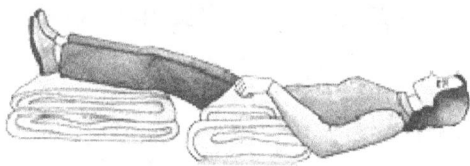

If the victim has a head wound or is having trouble breathing, elevate the *head and shoulders.* Do not elevate the feet and the head at the same time.

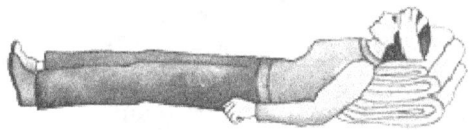

A victim who is bleeding from the mouth, vomiting, or may vomit should lie on one side, so fluid will drain from the mouth.

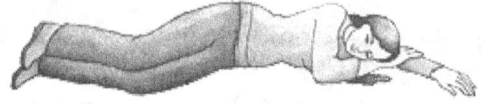

IF THE FACE IS RED RAISE THE HEAD
IF THE FACE IS PALE RAISE THE TAIL

Spinal injury:

If you suspect a back or neck (spinal) injury, do not move the affected person. Permanent paralysis and other serious complications can result. Assume a person has a spinal injury if:

- There's evidence of a head injury with an ongoing change in the person's level of consciousness

- The person complains of severe pain in his or her neck or back

- The person won't move his or her neck

- An injury has exerted substantial force on the back or head

- The person complains of weakness, numbness or paralysis or lacks control of his or her limbs, bladder or bowels

- The neck or back is twisted or positioned oddly

If you suspect someone has a spinal injury: Call 911 or emergency medical help.

- Keep the person still. Place heavy towels on both sides of the neck or hold the head and neck to prevent movement. The goal of first aid for a spinal injury is to keep the person in much the same position as he or she was found.

- Provide as much first aid as possible without moving the person's head or neck. If the person shows no signs of circulation (breathing, coughing or movement), begin CPR, but do not tilt the head back to open the airway. Use your fingers to gently grasp the jaw and lift it forward. If the person has no pulse, begin chest compressions.

- If the person is wearing a helmet, don't remove it.

- If you absolutely must roll the person because he or she is vomiting, choking on blood or in danger of further injury, you need at least one other person. With one of you at the head and another along the side of the injured person, work together to keep the person's head, neck and back aligned while rolling the person onto one side.

Stroke: (CVA)

A stroke occurs when there's bleeding into your brain or when normal blood flow to your brain is blocked. Within minutes of being deprived of essential nutrients, brain cells start dying — a process that may continue over the next several hours.

Seek immediate medical assistance. A stroke is a true emergency. The sooner treatment is given, the more likely it is that damage can be minimized. Every moment counts.

Signs and symptoms of a stroke include:

- Sudden weakness or numbness in your face, arm or leg on one side of your body

- Sudden dimness, blurring or loss of vision, particularly in one eye

- Loss of speech, trouble talking or understanding speech

- Sudden, severe headache — a bolt out of the blue — with no apparent cause

- Unexplained dizziness, unsteadiness or a sudden fall, especially if accompanied by any of the other signs or symptoms

Risk factors for stroke include having high blood pressure, having had a previous stroke, smoking, having diabetes and having heart disease. Your risk of stroke increases as you age.

Blank

Subconjunctival hemorrhage (broken blood vessel in eye)

A subconjunctival hemorrhage occurs when a tiny blood vessel breaks just underneath the clear surface of your eye (conjunctiva). You may not realize you have a subconjunctival hemorrhage until you look in the mirror and find the white part of your eye is bright red.

The conjunctiva can't absorb the blood quickly, so the blood is trapped under this transparent surface. A subconjunctival hemorrhage may look frightening and painful to you, but it's usually a harmless condition that disappears within 10 to 14 days.

Subconjunctival hemorrhage often occurs without any injury to your eye, or it may be the result of a strong sneeze or cough that caused a broken blood vessel. You don't need any specific treatment for a subconjunctival hemorrhage.

Symptoms

The most obvious sign of a subconjunctival hemorrhage is a bright red patch on the white (sclera) of the eye. Despite its bloody appearance, a subconjunctival hemorrhage should cause no change in your vision, no discharge from your eye and no pain. Your only discomfort may be a scratchy feeling on the surface of your eye.

When to see a doctor

If a bright red patch appears on your eye or on the eye of your child, contact your doctor to be sure that the problem is not more serious than a subconjunctival hemorrhage. If you have recurrent subconjunctival hemorrhages or other bleeding, talk to your doctor.

Causes

The cause of subconjunctival hemorrhage is usually unknown. However, the following actions may be enough to cause a small blood vessel to rupture in your eye:

- Violent coughing

- Powerful sneezing

- Heavy lifting

- Vomiting

Risk factors

People with diabetes or high blood pressure (hypertension) tend to be more at risk. The condition can also occur among newborns, who may be subjected to pressure changes during delivery.

Certain blood-thinning medications, such as warfarin and aspirin, can increase your risk of subconjunctival hemorrhage.

In addition, some herbal supplements, such as ginkgo, may increase the potential for bleeding in the eye. Be sure to tell your doctor if you're taking any herbal supplements.

While you may feel self-conscious about the appearance of your eye, health complications from a subconjunctival hemorrhage are rare.

The best way for your doctor or eye doctor (ophthalmologist) to diagnose subconjunctival hemorrhage is by looking at your eye. You'll likely need no other tests. However, your doctor may ask you some questions about your general health, take your blood pressure and obtain a routine blood test to make sure you don't have a potentially serious bleeding disorder.

You may want to use eyedrops, such as artificial tears, to soothe any scratchy feeling you have in your eye. Beyond that, the blood in your eye will absorb within 10 to 14 days and you'll need no further treatment.

WOUNDS:

Cuts and scrapes:

Minor cuts and scrapes usually don't require a trip to the emergency room. Yet proper care is essential to avoid infection or other complications. These guidelines can help you care for simple wounds:

1. **Stop the bleeding.** Minor cuts and scrapes usually stop bleeding on their own. If they don't, apply gentle pressure with a clean cloth or bandage. Hold the pressure continuously for 20 to 30 minutes and if possible elevate the wound. Don't keep checking to see if the bleeding has stopped because this may damage or dislodge the clot that's forming and cause bleeding to resume. If blood spurts or continues flowing after continuous pressure, seek medical assistance.

2. **Clean the wound.** Rinse out the wound with clear water. Soap can irritate the wound, so try to keep it out of the actual wound. If dirt or debris remains in the wound after washing, use tweezers cleaned with alcohol to remove the particles. If debris still remains, see your doctor. Thorough cleaning reduces the risk of infection and tetanus. To clean the area around the wound, use soap and a washcloth. There's no need to use hydrogen peroxide, iodine or an iodine-containing cleanser.

3. **Apply an antibiotic.** After you clean the wound, apply a thin layer of an antibiotic cream or ointment such as Neosporin or Polysporin to help keep the surface moist. The products don't make the wound heal faster, but they can discourage infection and help your body's natural healing process. Certain ingredients in some ointments can cause a mild rash in some people. If a rash appears, stop using the ointment.

4. **Cover the wound.** Bandages can help keep the wound clean and keep harmful bacteria out. After the wound has healed enough to make infection unlikely, exposure to the air will speed wound healing.

5. **Change the dressing.** Change the dressing at least daily or whenever it becomes wet or dirty. If you're allergic to the adhesive used in most

bandages, switch to adhesive-free dressings or sterile gauze held in place with paper tape, gauze roll or a loosely applied elastic bandage. These supplies generally are available at pharmacies.

6. **Get stitches for deep wounds.** A wound that is more than 1/4-inch (6 millimeters) deep or is gaping or jagged edged and has fat or muscle protruding usually requires stitches. Adhesive strips or butterfly tape may hold a minor cut together, but if you can't easily close the wound, see your doctor as soon as possible. Proper closure within a few hours reduces the risk of infection.

7. **Watch for signs of infection.** See your doctor if the wound isn't healing or you notice any redness, increasing pain, drainage, warmth or swelling.

8. **Get a tetanus shot.** Doctors recommend you get a tetanus shot every 10 years. If your wound is deep or dirty and your last shot was more than five years ago, your doctor may recommend a tetanus shot booster. Get the booster as soon as possible after the injury.

SKIN TREATMENT GUIDELINES

Pressure Ulcers to Ankles and Heels

WOUND   **Pressure ulcers to ankles and heels**

Definition   **All pressure ulcers to feet**

Possible
causes   *Friction – shearing - pressure*
_Or_
contributing
factors

Treatment   *Far any pressure ulcer to the feet DO NOT remove any eschar*
Guidelines   *or necrotic tissue. Cover with a dry dressing, change daily and*
                                PRN. Re-assess weekly for wound report

SKIN TREATMENT GUIDELINES

NUTRITION

Provide Substrates for Healing

It has long been recognized that protein is essential for wound repair and regeneration. Angiogenesis, fibroblast proliferation, collagen synthesis, and scar remodeling will not occur without essential amino acids. Amino acids are also necessary in supporting the immune response.

Because tissue injury results in increased protein metabolism and use of protein to promote wound healing, additional dietary sources are essential for patients with chronic wounds. Adequate amounts of fats and carbohydrates are needed in order to prevent the amino acids from being oxidized for caloric needs. Additionally glucose is needed to meet the energy requirements of the cells involved in wound repair.

Albumin

Albumin is the single most important indicator of malnutrition because it is sacrificed to provide essential amino acids in the event of inadequate protein intake. The half-life of albumin is 20 days therefore a low albumin is indicative of chronic malnourishment. Sporadic deficiencies in intake do not result in perceptible changes in serum albumin.

Lymphocytes

A lymphocyte count of less than 800 is another indicator of severe malnourishment. Nutritional supplementation should begin when the lymphocyte count is 1800.

Body Weight

Although inexpensive, body weight is of marginal value in detecting malnourishment.

Protein & Caloric Needs with Chronic Wounds

Protein Requirements = 1.25->1.5 Grams of protein per kg of body weight per day

Caloric Requirements = 30 - 35 calories per kg of body weight per day. If the person is unable maintain an adequate food intake high nutrient supplements should be used to meet the nutritional needs.

Necessary Vitamin and Mineral Supplementation & Wound Healing

> **Vitamin A -> Multivitamin daily**
> **B Vitamins -> Multivitamin daily**
> **Vitamin C -> Multivitamin daily**
> **Zinc -> 220-mg/ day in presence of deficiency**
> **Iron -> Supplement only if no active infection**

SKIN TREATMENT GUIDELINES

WOUND   **Excoriation/Denuded Skin**

Definition   **Skin alteration resulting in reddened area with loss of**
epidermis.

Possible
causes   *Scratches – skin infection – fungal growth – scraping or rubbing*
_Or_   **friction burns**
contributing
factors

Treatment   *Cleanse area with soap and water*
Guidelines   **Reduce cause – trim nails, treat infection as ordered**
                       Use transfer device to reduce friction.
                       Obtain order for physician recommended cream to excoriated
                       area B.I.D and P.R.N

SKIN TREATMENT GUIDELINES

WOUND	**Rash**
Definition	**Skin eruption from a multitude of causes**
Possible causes *Or* *contributing* *factors*	*Allergic reaction – Scabies – Yeast infection - dermatitis*
Treatment Guidelines	*Notify physician and describe appearance, location if it itches the resident, and any new medications and or treatments that the resident is on.* **Obtain order for P.O. Benadryl 25 – 50 mg q 6hrs prn Times 10 days or until gone, or other medication as ordered By the physician.**

SKIN TREATMENT GUIDELINES

WOUND	**Skin Tear**
Definition	**Skin Alteration resulting in loss of epidermis or more, with or Without a skin flap**
Possible causes *Or* contributing factors	*Advanced age with subsequent thin, frail, skin* dehydration
Treatment Guidelines or	*Cleanse with saline to help with approximation if needed. Approximate flap and secure with steri strips. Apply* **Small amount of TAO and cover with Telfa dressing and Tape**

Wrap with Kerlex to secure.
Obtain order for; Apply small amount of TAO and cover with Telfa dressing and Tape or Wrap with Kerlex to secure, Q day Times Two weeks or until healed.

If skin around area becomes macerated, obtain order to D/C TAO.
If wound will not dry up and heal, obtain order to D/C TAO And cover with dry dressing, or other treatment as ordered by the physician.

SKIN TREATMENT GUIDELINES

WOUND	**Blister**
Definition	**Small or large raised lesion filled with fluid**
Possible causes _Or_ _contributing_ _factors_	*Friction – Burn – Allergic reaction*
Treatment Guidelines	*If blister is intact – cover blister with tegaderm* *If blister is open – treat as skin tear (see skin tear guidelines)* **If blister is in buttocks or in the peri area where soiling may occur, cover with telfa and tegaderm.**

SKIN TREATMENT GUIDELINES

WOUND   Stage I

Definition   Any area of redness on light skin OR red, blue or
                             purple on darker skin. Persistent redness is determined
                             only after
                             Pressure has been relieved at least ½ - ¾ of the time it
was

                             Applied to cause the redness.

Possible causes   *Pressure – incontinence - Friction*
Or
contributing
factors

Treatment   *Pressure relieving devices (air mattress – Gel cushion)*
Guidelines   *Avoid shearing when moving*
                             Turn and reposition Q2hrs and PRN
                             Barrier Cream to area Q shift and PRN

SKIN TREATMENT GUIDELINES

WOUND   Stage II

Definition   Skin loss involving dermis, epidermis or both. Ulcer is
superficial

Possible causes   *Friction – shearing - pressure*
Or
contributing
factors

Treatment   *Obtain order to Assess Albumin level if <3.5 notify physician for*
Guidelines   *Promod or Arginaid, zinc, and Vit C*
                              DO NOT use donut type devices
                              When up in chair, reposition Q1hr and PRN
                              If alert and oriented encourage to shift weight q 15 min
                              When in bed reposition Q2 hrs
                              Cleanse wound Q shift and PRN with normal saline
                              Apply barrier cream
                              If it is not draining cover with tegaderm
                              If there is light drainage cover with a hydrcolloid
                              If there is moderate drainage cover with a foam dressing

                              If the resident is having frequent diarrhea, do not cover wound
                              As it may harbor infection
                              Clean after each stool and apply Baza or other barrier, or
                              other treatment as ordered by the physician

SKIN TREATMENT GUIDELINES

WOUND	**Stage III**
Definition	**A full thickness of skin is lost.(epidermal layer has been lost exposing the subcutaneous tissues) presents a shallow crater unless covered by eschar – thick brown, black, or yellow crust. May be draining**
Possible causes _Or_ _contributing factors_	_Pressure – infection Poor circulation_
Treatment	_Prevent infection, remove necrotic tissue, cover – insulate – and hydrate. Obliterate dead space, promote granulation._
Guidelines	**Select dressing that Controls exudates but does not dry wound.**
Nutrition **supplement**	**Monitor intake, MVI with minerals, vitamin C, Zinc, 8oZ of milk with each meal if tolerated, Eval for**
LAB's	_CBC, BMP, Albumin level if < 3.5, give Promod or_ **Arginaid**
Equipment	_Pressure relieving devices, Heel protectors_

SKIN TREATMENT GUIDELINES

WOUND	Stage IV
Definition	Full thickness of skin and subcutaneous tissue is lost. Exposing muscle and/or bone; this sore may be covered with eschar, draining, necrotic, reddened, and/or indurated.
Possible causes Or *contributing factors*	*Excess pressure, Poor care, poor circulation.*
Treatment	*Prevent infection, remove necrotic tissue, cover (except wounds to heels and ankles) – insulate – and hydrate. Obliterate dead space, promote granulation.*
Guidelines	*Select dressing that Controls exudates but does not dry wound. Moisten when needed apply absorption when needed*
Nutrition	Monitor intake, MVI with minerals, vitamin C, Zinc, 8oz of milk with each meal if tolerated, Eval for supplement
LAB's	CBC, BMP, Albumin level if < 3.5, give Promod or Arginaid
Equipment	Pressure relieving devices, Heel protectors

blank

99

Blank

100

Basic Life Support

Cardio-Pulmonary Respiration

1. **Stay Safe!** The worst thing a rescuer can do is become another victim. Follow universal precautions and wear personal protective equipment if you have it. Use common sense and stay away from potential hazards.

2. **Attempt to wake victim**. Briskly rub your knuckles against the victim's sternum. If the victim does not wake, **call 911** and proceed to step 3. If the victim wakes, moans, or moves, then CPR is not necessary at this time. Call 911 if the victim is confused or not able to speak.

3. **Begin rescue breathing**. Open the victim's airway using the head-tilt, chin-lift method. Put your ear to the victim's open mouth:

   - look for chest movement
   - listen for air flowing through the mouth or nose
   - feel for air on your cheek

   If there is no breathing, pinch the victim's nose; make a seal over the victim's mouth with yours. Use a CPR mask if available. Give the victim a breath big enough to make the chest rise. Let the chest fall, then repeat the rescue breath once more. If the chest doesn't rise on the first breath, reposition the head and try again. Whether it works on the second try or not, go to step 4.

4. **Begin chest compressions**. Place the heel of your hand in the middle of the victim's chest. Put your other hand on top of the first with your fingers interlaced. Compress the chest about 1-1/2 to 2 inches (4-5 cm). Allow the chest to completely recoil before the next compression. Compress the chest at a rate equal to 100/minute. Perform 30 compressions at this rate.

5. **Repeat rescue breaths**. Open the airway with head-tilt, chin-lift again. This time, go directly to rescue breaths without checking for breathing again. Give one breath, making sure the chest rises and falls, then give another. Remember, if the chest doesn't rise on the first breath, reposition the head before you give the second breath.

6.   **Perform 30 more chest compressions**. Repeat steps 5 and 6 for about two minutes.

7.   After 2 minutes of chest compressions and rescue breaths, stop compressions and recheck victim for breathing. If the victim is not breathing, continue chest compressions and rescue breaths.

8.   Keep going until help arrives.

Tips:

1.   If you have acces to an automated external defibrillator, attach it to the victim after approximately one minute of CPR (chest compressions and rescue breaths).

2.   Chest compressions are extremely important. If you are not comfortable giving rescue breaths, still perform chest compressions!

3.   It's normal to feel pops and snaps when you first begin chest compressions - DON'T STOP! You aren't going to make the victim any worse. Cardiac arrest is as bad as it gets.

4.   When performing chest compressions, do not let your hands bounce. Let the chest fully recoil, but keep the heel of your hand in contact with the sternum at all times.

5.   For more information on these steps go to the Emergency Cardiac Care (ECC) Guidelines from the American Heart Association.

1. CALL

Check the victim for unresponsiveness. If there is no response, Call 911 and return to the victim. In most locations the emergency dispatcher can assist you with CPR instructions.

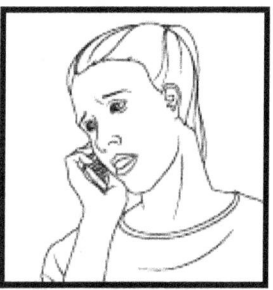

2. BLOW

Tilt the head back and listen for breathing. If not breathing normally, pinch nose and cover the mouth with yours and blow until you see the chest rise. Give 2 breaths. Each breath should take 1 second.

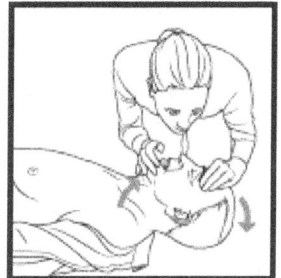

3. PUMP

If the victim is still not breathing normally, coughing or moving, begin chest compressions. Push down on the chest 1½ to 2 inches 30 times right between the nipples. Pump at the rate of 100/minute, faster than once per second.

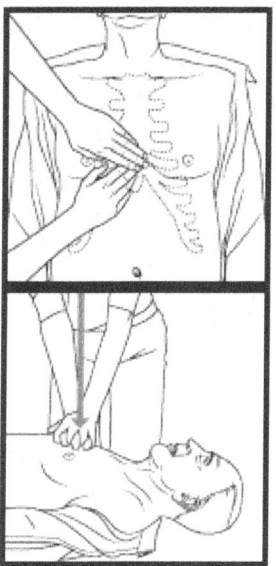

The Heimlich Maneuver® for CHOKING ADULTS

A choking victim can't speak or breathe and needs your help immediately. Follow these steps to help a choking victim:

1. From behind, wrap your arms around the victim's waist.
2. Make a fist and place the thumb side of your fist against the victim's upper abdomen, below the ribcage and above the navel.
3. Grasp your fist with your other hand and press into their upper abdomen with a quick upward thrust. Do not squeeze the ribcage; confine the force of the thrust to your hands.
4. Repeat until object is expelled.

UNCONSCIOUS VICTIM, OR WHEN RESCUER CAN'T REACH AROUND VICTIM:
Place the victim on back. Facing the victim, kneel astride the victim's hips. With one of your hands on top of the other, place the heel of your bottom hand on the upper abdomen below the rib cage and above the navel. Use your body weight to press into the victim's upper abdomen with a quick upward thrust. Repeat until object is expelled. If the Victim has not recovered, proceed with CPR.
The Victim should see a physician immediately after rescue.

Don't slap the victim's back. (This could make matters worse.)

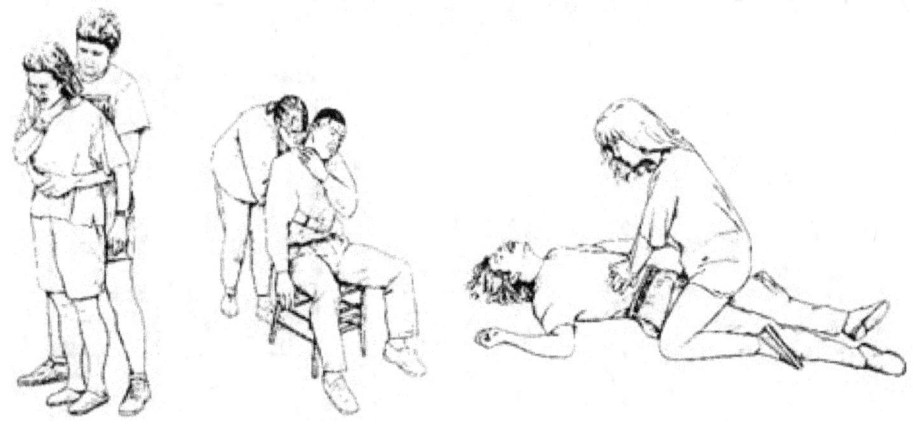

The Heimlich Maneuver for CHOKING INFANTS

A choking victim can't speak or breathe and needs your help immediately.

Follow these steps to help a choking infant:

Lay the child down, face up, on a firm surface and kneel or stand at the victim's feet, or hold infant on your lap facing away from you. Place the middle and index fingers of both your hands below his rib cage and above his navel. Press into the victim's upper abdomen with a quick upward thrust; do not squeeze the rib cage. Be very gentle. Repeat until object is expelled.

If the Victim has not recovered, proceed with CPR. The Victim should see a physician immediately after rescue.

Don't slap the victim's back. (This could make matters worse.)

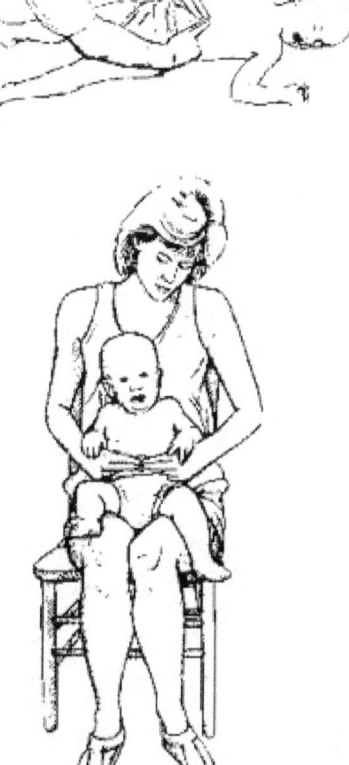

The Heimlich Maneuver for CHOKING (ONESELF)

When you choke, you can't speak or breathe and you need help immediately. Follow these steps to save yourself from choking:

1. Make a fist and place the thumb side of your fist against your upper abdomen, below the ribcage and above the navel.
2. Grasp your fist with your other hand and press into your upper abdomen with a quick upward thrust.
3. Repeat until object is expelled.

Alternatively, you can lean over a fixed horizontal object (table edge, chair, railing) and press your upper abdomen against the edge to produce a quick upward thrust. Repeat until object is expelled.

See a physician immediately after rescue.

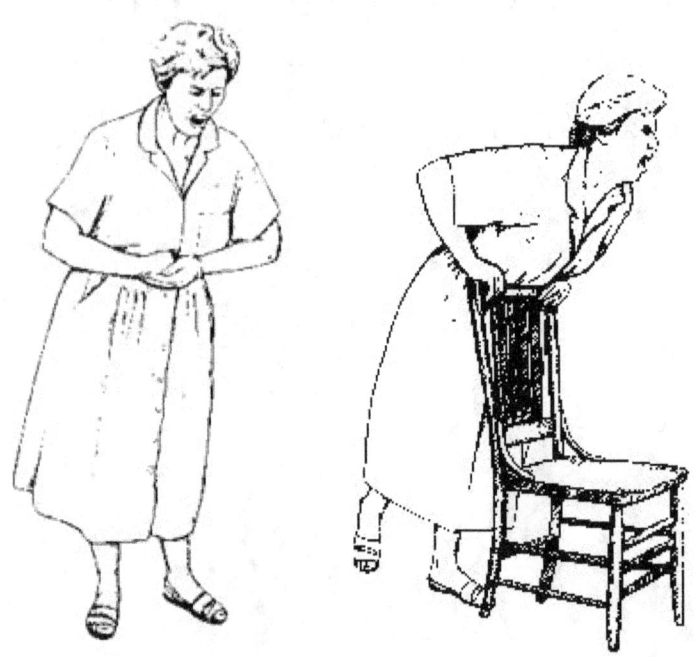

BABYSITTING INFORMATION SHEET

ADDRESS OF SITTING_____

NEAREST CROSS STREETS_____

MOTHERS NAME_____CELL _____

FATHERS NAME_____CELL_____

OTHER CONTACT_____PHONE_____

CHILDS NAME_____AGE_____

FOOD ALLERGIES_____

MEDICATION ALLERGIES_____

NEED TO KNOW_____

_____

CHILDS NAME_____AGE_____

FOOD ALLERGIES_____

MEDICATION ALLERGIES_____

NEED TO KNOW_____

_____

For printable version of this form and other caregiving forms visit my web site where they can be downloaded www.lighthouseseniorservices.com or email me and I will email you one back at kennedy@lighthouseseniorservices.com

With each new client OR new location have the family fill this out. INSIST on it. You only have to do it once then the next time you baby sit just bring this with. To make sure that the parents have time to fill it out, the first time you sit for them, arrive 5 minutes early so they can complete it. Nobody wants an emergency, but the only way to handle one is to be prepared.

About the Author

Charles Kennedy RN, LNHA, CSSC.
Author, nurse and Founder of Lighthouse Senior Services. Has been a registered nurse since 1982.
 For almost 30 years his focus has been in geriatric care.
His work in both Skilled Nursing facilities as a Director of Nursing and Licensed Nursing Home Administrator. As well as a Director of Operations in the Home Health arena, has offered him the unique opportunity to understand the needs and frustrations of so many seniors and their loved ones.
Charles can be contacted at kennedy@lighthouseseniorservices.com
Visit him at www.lighthouseseniorservices.com

NOTES

www.ingramcontent.com/pod-product-compliance
Lightning Source LLC
Chambersburg PA
CBHW081358280526
45788CB00009B/2915